HOLY COW
I HAVE CANCER!

NOW WHAT?

DAVID W. SCHELL, ED.D.

ACKNOWLEDGMENTS

Literally hundreds of people have been lovingly involved in my journey with cancer and the creation of this book. These include friends, loved ones, caregivers and prayer groups. To list each one would be a mammoth task.

However, I would like to acknowledge the contributions of my two brothers: Dr. John Schell, who provided invaluable assistance and photographs and D.R. Schell (Dan), who served as a contributing editor. Also Brad Schell (John's son), who rescued us from terrible technological nightmares. This book is offered in a spirit of love from the "Rough and Tumble" Schell boys.

- David W. Schell, Ed.D.

FORWARD

Further along we'll know all about it,
Further along we'll understand why;
Cheer up my brother, live in the sunshine,
We'll understand it all by and by.

- Traditional American Hymn

Why does David have life-threatening cancer? I have no earthly idea. His faith assures that further along he'll understand why. But, is he waiting for a big heavenly revelation? Not on your life. This narrative represents his experiences – his lived experiences. David is making meaning and seeking answers to questions that are posed just beyond our human understanding.

David, our middle brother Dan, and I come from a Missouri working class family where hard work and effort are revered and expected. As the oldest David set that standard for the Schell boys. He made sure that Dan and I hoed all of those tomatoes while he supervised from the shade.

Now, however, we are coming to the ends of our youth and careers. David especially is facing a rising flood of health concerns that prevent him from exercising his lifelong philosophy: Work hard; play even harder. Cancer is little by little transforming his identity. It is a cruel twist of fate for David; definitely NOT what he had in mind for retirement.

In this brief narrative he shares his deepest thoughts and feelings with a sense of honesty and "pulls no punches." He is giving this narrative as a gift to those who have or will travel along a similar road. These thoughts, feelings and insights are his way of giving you and members of your family needed comfort, support and understanding.

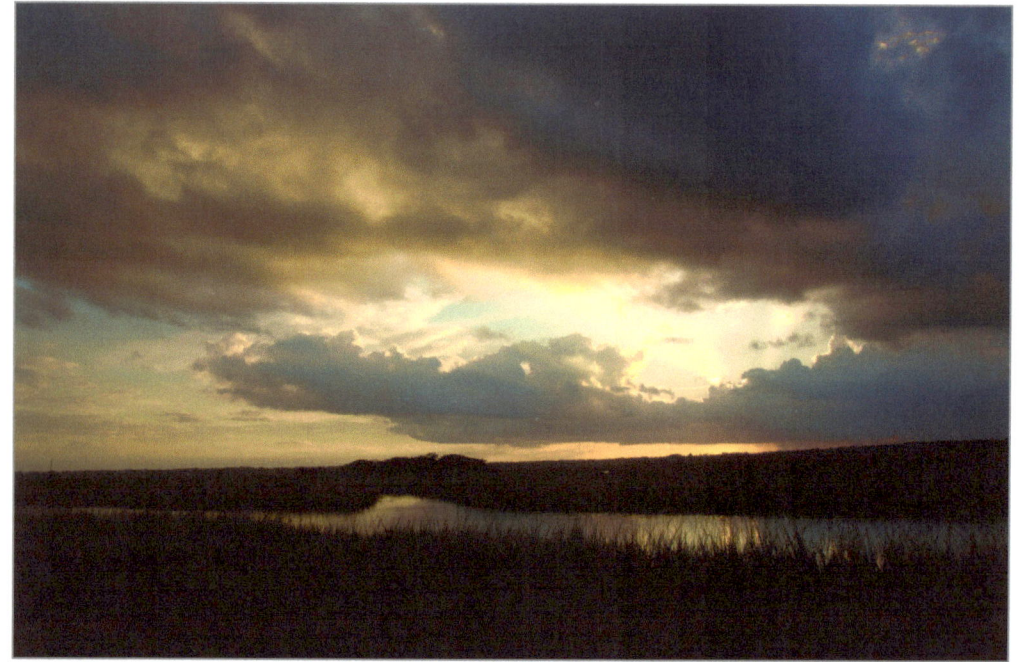

Picture in Memory of Zela Schell

You will read of David's joys and accomplishments. But you will also read about the reality of his heartbreak, personal anger, frustration, and bitter arguments with his God.

Yet, if you were to call him on the telephone today he would greet you enthusiastically and ask about your health long before he might admit to feeling gimpy. I love this about my brother. He lives in the sunshine and shares it with all of us.

In no way will his cancer defeat him. He may not survive it, but his spirit will never be defeated by an illness. If he has to face death, he will do it with dignity and grace… a life well lived. That is who he always has been, is and who he will be.

When the time comes to part from this earth we will say the same simple words that we speak at the end of each visit or phone call: "I love you, bro!"

- John W. Schell, Ph.D.
Professor Emeritus
University of Georgia

SUDDEN CRISIS

JANUARY, 2010

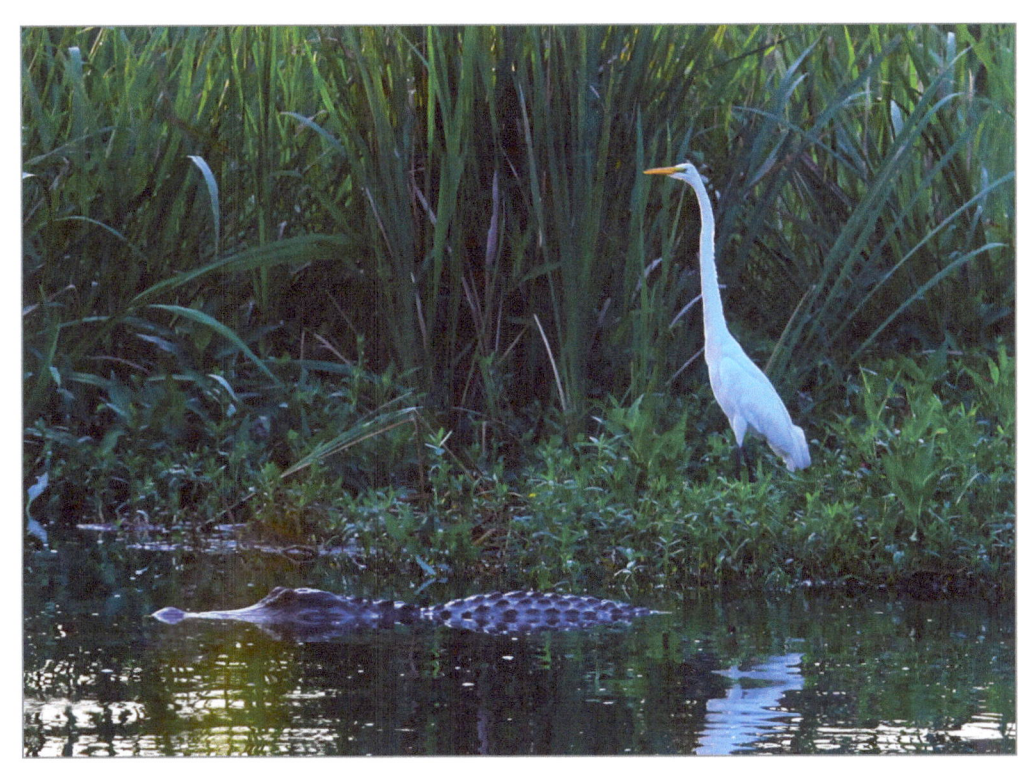

Feeling fine. Mark of health. Walking 2-3 miles a day. Bang! Sudden diagnosis of B-Cell Lymphoma and Stage 4 Colon cancer. Choices narrowed down to immediate surgery and months or a lifetime of chemotherapy or die within the next six months. Yes, I said, "die" as in dead—caput! I have seen a lot of death during my lifetime, but this is MY death! My soul cries out in denial and confusion.

Angry? What was I to do? Jump up and down and yell "Yippee I have cancer!" If I was not a particularly angry person before, I found myself enraged over my diagnoses, sudden collapse of my profession, and related physical limitations. Angry at God? Oh, yes. I may as well admit it. After all He knows it anyway. Who do I think I am fooling?

Some of my friends are shocked over my being angry with God and tell me it is His will. That is about as comforting as a splinter in my eye. I found myself shouting at God, letting Him know in no uncertain terms what I think of his will. I used a few strong words we don't normally hear in church or in polite company. Yet, I believe He fully understood the depth of my rampage. I know God's will supersedes mine. After all, He could smash me like a bloated dog tick. I felt bullied. I have been warned that such thoughts may be blasphemous. Maybe so, but my feelings were real and ready to explode like Mt. St. Helens. I recalled the words of Dylan Thomas who wrote, "Do not go gentle into that good night. . . Rage, rage against the dying of light".

For thirty-seven years I had enjoyed a fulfilling career as a Licensed Professional Counselor and a Marriage and Family Therapist. I had built a successful practice and became accustomed to providing therapy for those in need. My office was adorned with what one of my colleagues calls an "I love me wall", complete with degrees, licensures, certifications and recognitions. One advantage to my "I love me wall" (aside from filling legal requirements to practice) is that it affirmed my identity, at least professionally. Of course one does not need a display of credentials to have a healthy sense of personal identity and direction. But inevitably, the question came, "Now who am I?" I looked the same in the mirror, but I felt lost and useless.

In addition to my professional practice, I provided years of caregiving for my wife who suffered long term agonizing pain before she lost her courageous battle with bladder cancer. Now I ask myself, am I a caregiver or a caregivee?

Soon after my diagnosis, I began to experience the, "Why Me Syndrome". Why am I being punished? What did I do to deserve this? Chemotherapy made me sick and weak. Is it worth going on? "Why Me" partners easily with "Poor Me". Memories of my wife's unfair anguish rushed back into vivid consciousness. I found myself hammered by medication, discouraged by depression, limited by physical weakness, fear, and besieged by uncertainty and loss of control. Eventually, I ventured to ask myself, "Why Not Me?" Why did she die in spite of being a beautiful person and having the best care available? I began to realize that cancer is no respecter of persons. I began to wonder if God is that way too. Darned if I know.

Now all of a sudden I am the one in need of care. I reluctantly gave up my fulfilling practice. After all, my clients deserved more than a therapist with Eloxatin, FU5, Avastin, and a host of other medications sloshing around in my brain in tandem with my own fears, frustrations, depression and anger.

My "I Love Me" wall no longer seemed so important. However, I have left it in place and strive to maintain my credentials. The wall now serves as an apple on a stick encouraging me to regain my health and return to active practice.

In the hospital while waiting on a gurney for scans, I struck up a conversation with a man on a gurney next to me. He had been severely injured in a motorcycle accident and could not feel anything from his neck down. We chatted and tried to encourage one another.

My scans confirmed cancer had spread throughout my body. Strangely enough, I thought I could feel heat from the lesions as my body passed through one of those big scary marvels of technology. I found myself wallowing in anger and self-pity as I was subjected to riding through a big mechanical doughnut called an MRI. I was half way through the doughnut when all of a sudden an inner voice came to me saying, "David, you have forgotten to be grateful".

Mea Culpa. I had become self-centered. Nothing seemed to matter but my own health, situation and circumstances. I recalled the man in the next gurney who may never walk again. I had walked into the hospital and had every expectation of walking out. I found myself silently praying for my hospital companion.

I don't claim to have special access to God, but I believe the MRI experience was His way of speaking to me. I felt I was offered a compass to plot my course through the labyrinth of anger, confusion and uncertainty. Nothing mysterious, but nevertheless a spiritual experience. Crazy? Maybe. But it was a turning point for me. An answer? No, just a turning point. Is God pushing me around or am I hearing the comfort of a "still small voice"? I would have preferred a GPS to a compass.

After the MRI experience, I began to think in more positive directions. I could not see or know my final destiny with cancer, but at least I had a compass. I felt my body begin to relax. I had forgotten who had given me life in the first place. I was being provided with the best medical attention available. Doctors who did not know me had gone to extraordinary lengths to assure I was provided with immediate lifesaving procedures. How was it these particular doctors were there when, unbeknownst to me, I desperately needed their lifesaving skills? Could it be that God put these people in the right place at the right time? Go figure! I came to realize my anger toward God is not synonymous with alienation. His love is not diminished by my raging anger. I emerged from the MRI in a state of prayerful gratitude.

Many friends and family have extended needed emotional and spiritual support. Several churches continue to hold me up to God's throne of grace. Individual "prayer warriors" faithfully pray for my recovery. I have learned that support is immediate and helps build a foundation for comfort and resolution that may come in time. In the meantime, their support brings strength and encouragement. I may have stage 4 cancer, but I am a wealthy man.

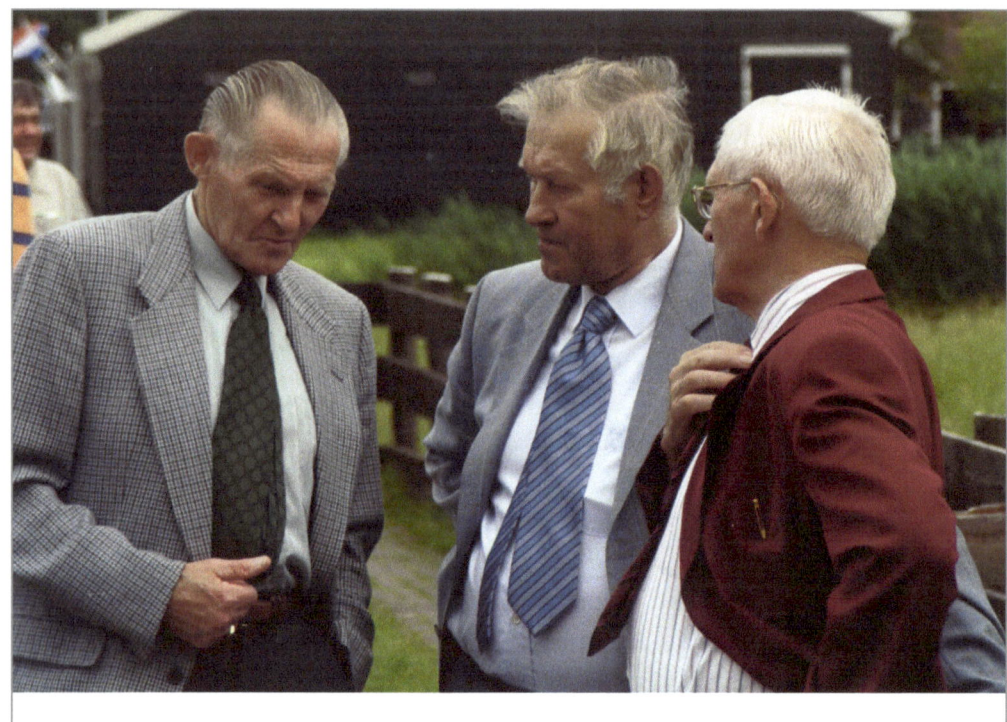

Friends with the best intentions come offering advice. I think of Job in the
Bible (check it out, it is in the Old Testament) whose well-meaning comforters
attempted to help him understand why his life had turned from gold to total
disaster. Seems to me, Job had the Midas touch in reverse. My suffering does
not begin to approach the suffering of Job, but I can relate to the advice of his
comforters. Most biblical scholars are critical of these comforters. But I think
that is unfair. I believe their hearts were in the right place even if their advice
was about as useful as a sidesaddle on a pig.

Like Job, I have collected and listened to the sage advice of many well-meaning
friends who trot out numerous cases involving friends, relatives, and associates
who are cited as examples of healing. I call this the "Aunt Tilley and Uncle Toad
Phenomena". For instance some tell me if I have enough faith I will be healed.
That sure worked for Aunt Tilley. Yes, I pray to be healed and work diligently to
that end. But if I am not healed, the implication is a lack of faith. I don't buy that.
Still others believe cancer is evil and I must rid myself of the evil, which is causing
the disease. I am told such things as Uncle Toad gave up smokin' drinkin' and
dancin' and lived another 20 years. Well duh! We are all evil. Why aren't we all

Holy Cow! I Have CANCER! Now What?

eaten up with cancer? Some professional friends suggest I use meditation or creative imagery or some popular New Age techniques. I do these things but if I am not healed, does that mean I am psychologically or spiritually inadequate? I don't buy that either. A few friends have suggested I am being tested. Tested for what? Why would God test me? I believe God and I are reasonably aware of my strengths and weaknesses. One of my favorite gems is that I need to eat more carrots. This might work. I have been told flamingos are sometimes fed carrots until they turn pink. Come to think of it, I have never heard of or seen a pink flamingo with colon cancer.

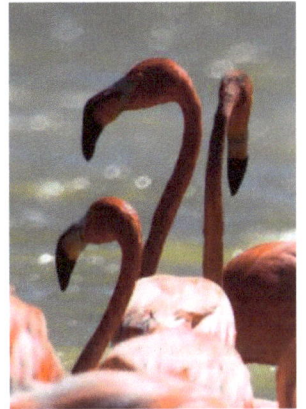

To be sure, my well-meaning comforters have my best interest at heart. I love them for their intentions rather than being irritated at their goofy advice.

Although I am a realist, I have learned to laugh and enjoy life in the midst of uncertainty. My father once commented that death is as natural as birth. I cannot afford to indulge in self-pity and negativistic thinking. Maintaining a sense of optimism is important. However, a Pollyanna approach to optimism often overlooks reality. I am reminded of the little girl who proclaimed, "I don't stink because I am a Christian".

Realistically, I have learned those who die suddenly may be spared protracted suffering but usually their families bear the acute brunt of that loss. Those who die gradually have opportunities to prepare themselves, their friends and their families. Many of us who suffer cancer have that opportunity.

I love life and have been very fortunate, which makes the idea of losing my life especially difficult. However, I have discovered that I may have a bad attitude and be miserable or a good attitude and be at peace. I may not control the outcome of my cancer, but I can control my attitude and the quality of my journey. Are these coping mechanisms? Probably, but I don't care to give them up. Humor and realistic positive thinking make my friends and loved ones feel better too. Sure beats doom and gloom.

David Schell © 2011

In the final analysis, I have learned each person must work out his or her own way of coping with major crises in life. We might learn something from Aunt Tilly and Uncle Toad, but when all is said and done, each of us must find our own way. God has given us the ability to do just that. Yet, only a fool does not consider the advice and guidance of others. Fortunately, there are spiritual and physical resources available to all of us. I recall getting lost in the sky while training for my private pilot's license. I did not know which way to go, but I had a compass and a heading indicator. Following the directions of my flight instructor and learning to read the instruments got us safely home.

No two of us are alike, but we can learn from each other.

At the time of this writing my brain is saturated with heavy doses of chemotherapy. But perhaps a few useful pearls will float to the top. With that in mind, I share a concept that has been helpful to me. I call the concept, "Let Go and Let God. . ."

Notice I placed an ellipsis at the end. The ellipsis represents the unknown. Should I "let go and let God"; I really don't know what will happen. I am faced with even more uncertainties. I am confronted with a journey that can have life or death consequences. That is pretty scary. I feel something like Ulysses facing the Cyclops.

Okay, So Now What?

February, 2010

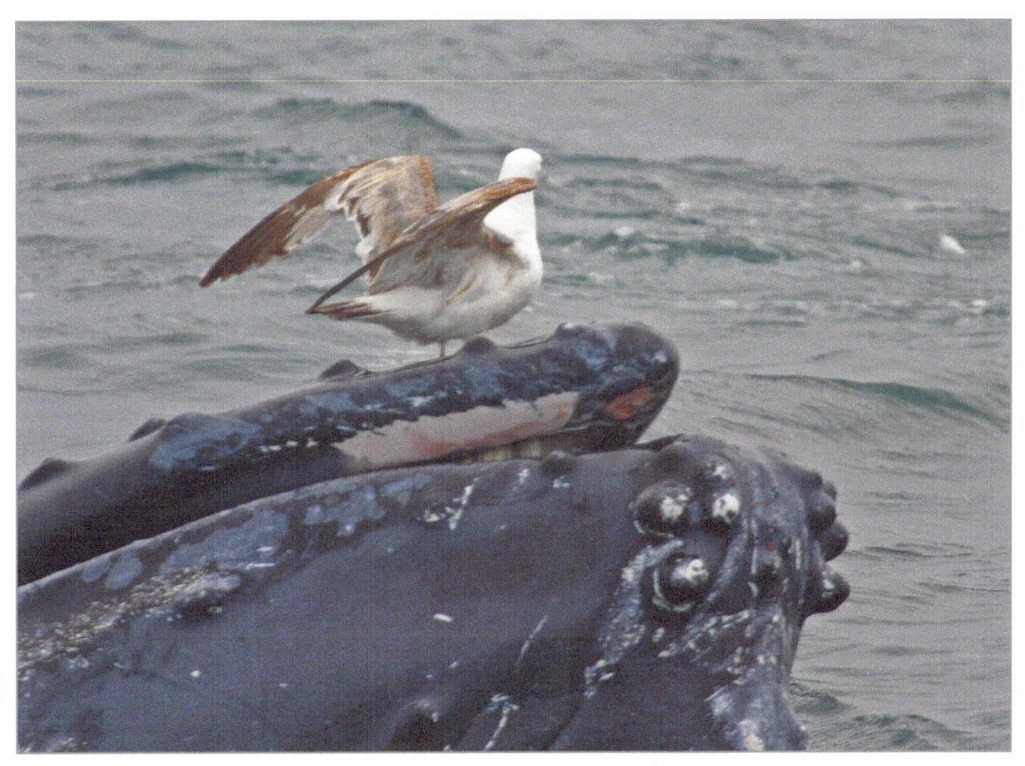

The "letting go" sounds simple enough. But for a control freak like me it is difficult. The "letting God" is even more difficult. This entails turning my life and destiny over to a God I have never seen and who may well be enraged at me. I don't even know which church He attends. I think this is called faith.

For me the uncertainty is the most complicated. I study the statistics and find I will likely live a little longer. Not as long as I had hoped, but longer than my first fears indicated. But who knows, tomorrow I could be run over by a truck. Sometimes life seems like a pinball machine. To be sure, eventually each ball drops down a hole. I recall as children we used to chant, "Yes, no, maybe so". Pursuing the meaning of the rest of my life brings back that same feeling of uncertainty.

I know my will. My will is to be healed and resume my life. After all, God gave us the natural will to live. We are endowed with survival skills. On the other hand, I don't know what God's will might be regarding my cancer and the rest of my life. What if He chooses to let me die? I have seen that happen to better people than me. What if I must pay for all the rotten things I have done in life? Now that can get really scary. Yet, somehow I hear the voice of God echo through the centuries as He advised St. Paul, "My grace is sufficient for thee". Well, I am no St. Paul, but I believe His grace is greater than the anger I have experienced.

Perhaps God may spare my life for a specific purpose. Today, as I write, I have no idea what that purpose might be. My purpose seems all tied up with the uncertainty of my journey with cancer. My brother, who is an accomplished professor, reminded me we don't have to have a title to have purpose. Some years ago, I learned that one does not have to wait for specific directions. Let me illustrate the point.

During my graduate studies, I was able to train in an acute care mental hospital. My professors were wise and graciously shared their wisdom, knowledge and experiences with me. My work in the hospital was exhausting but rewarding. I recall meeting with my major professor toward the end of a particularly grueling semester. For clarification, I reminded him he had never given me specific requirements for that particular semester. I was anxious, as I knew I would be graded on the quality of my work.

My professor thought a moment before speaking. In a serious tone, he said, "David, here are the requirements. You grab a shovel and dig. The needs in this hospital are so great; it matters little where you dig. Wherever you dig you will find need and someone who needs your help." I got an A for that semester. But more importantly, I have never forgotten his insights and sage advice. Today, I am learning that cancer is no excuse. Yes, God may have a specific direction or tasks for our lives, but when we are uncertain, human needs are so great, we can always grab a shovel and dig.

In my trek with cancer, I question, does God lead or direct individuals to certain tasks? I think of Jonah, who resisted his God given assignment and ended up in a blob of whale puke regurgitated on a shore near Nineveh. Whales exhale through blowholes located in the top of their heads. If you have ever smelled the stench of whale breath, you will take this lesson seriously.

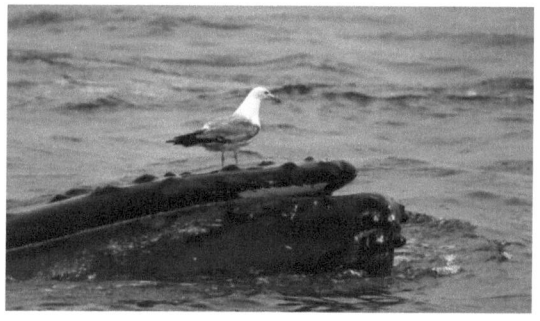

Recently, I had a long distance telephone conversation with a beloved cousin who was nearing the premature end of her life. She knew she was dying but exhibited a beautiful attitude that encouraged me. Her love and caring extended beyond herself. Strange, I called to comfort her. She had found and made peace with her journey. I thought maybe I could make peace with my journey too. A few days later she passed on, leaving me a legacy of inner strength. Maybe in some way, I can follow her example of courage and fearless faith.

Where is my journey with cancer taking me? I don't know. That is in His hands. Today, I see through a glass darkly. Sometimes that glass is so dark I wonder if a crystal ball might tell me more. Nevertheless, I have learned that faith; hope and love are core values for life no matter how long we live or how much we suffer. I suspect these values extend beyond life as we know it.

When my lymphoma and cancer were first diagnosed and after surgery, I was told without treatment I might have six more months to live. My own research affirmed this prognosis. It also affirmed my oncologist was on the leading edge of colon cancer treatment. Obviously, I elected to undergo chemotherapy. Today, I am alive and having a lot of good days. While my oncologist does not talk about recovery or cure, he is optimistic about controlling my cancer. Some days the chemotherapy makes me sick. On those "bad days" I have learned to thank God, as feeling bad is also a signal the medication is working in my body.

A Big Bump in the Road

July, 2010

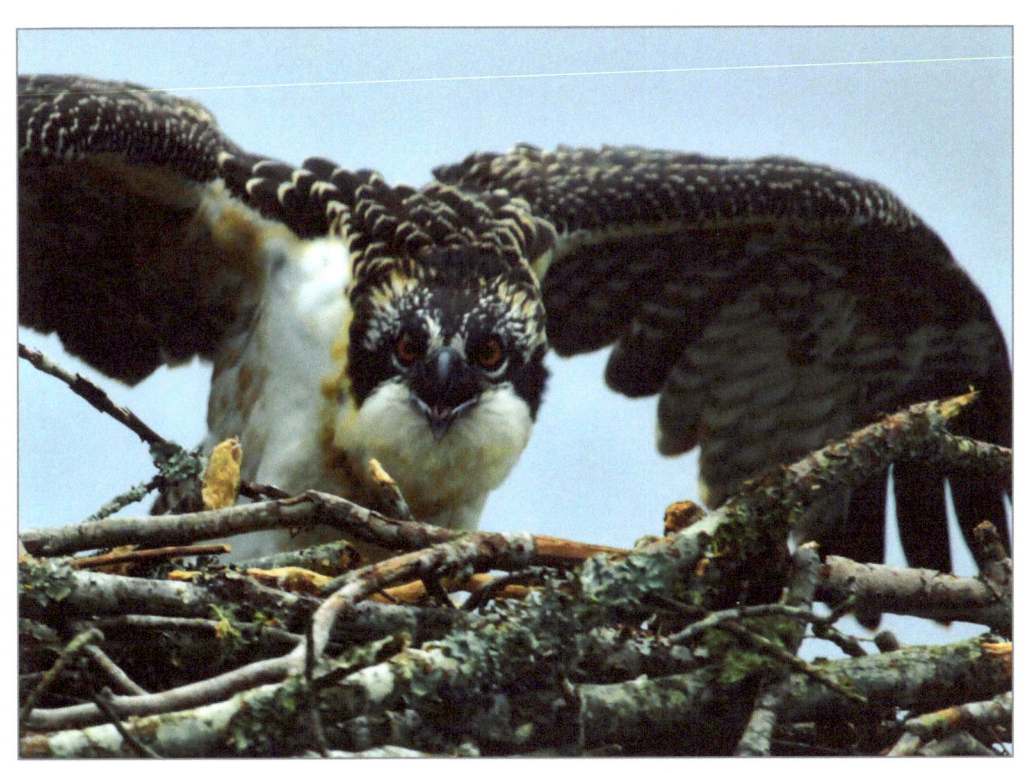

Bang! Again. My journey suddenly became even more complicated. I began experiencing chest pains and sweating. Could it be? No, surely not. I described these symptoms to my oncologist who immediately stopped my chemotherapy. The next thing I knew I was sitting in the office of a cardiologist.

My denial system weakened as I watched the cardiologist's face become grim when I described how both my mother and my father had heart bypasses when they were about my age. He scheduled me immediately for an EKG, and echocardiogram, and a stress test.

Stress test? In a jocular manner I protested, "Of course I am stressed". My lame attempt at humor brought a polite smile and lightened the intensity of the moment for both of us. He was a little less grim; I was a little less stressed. Though serious, my new cardiologist and I were on the same wavelength. But my cancer journey had suddenly become more complicated. My destination became even more uncertain.

My chemo-soaked brain raced desperately for any explanation other than heart trouble. After all, the chest pains may be no more than gastric distress, or the side effects of chemotherapy, or as serious as a heart attack. I can't ever remember praying for gas pains. Now I prayed in earnest these pains might be cured by simple flatulence. I ventured to wonder if God would smile at such a request.

During the echo cardiogram the technician positioned me so I could see my own heart beating. I was dumbfounded with the amazement as I watched my heart valves open and close with tireless synchrony. I was stunned at the intricacies of God's creation. This tiny part of His creation was for no other purpose than to give ME life. I recalled the first words of Samuel Morse's telegraph, "What hath God wrought?" Again I found gratitude in the midst of human technology. I pondered; If God's grace is as profound as His creation, there is hope beyond my journey with cancer.

New hope indeed. After an anxious twenty-four hour wait, the results of my heart tests came back. My heart looked strong and even younger than my age. Yes, God seemed to have smiled on my request for a flatulent cure for my thoracic distress. My oncologist also smiled and affirmed such cures for early heart disease are not uncommon. He resumed my chemotherapy.

Where Am I Going and How Do I Get There?

August, 2010

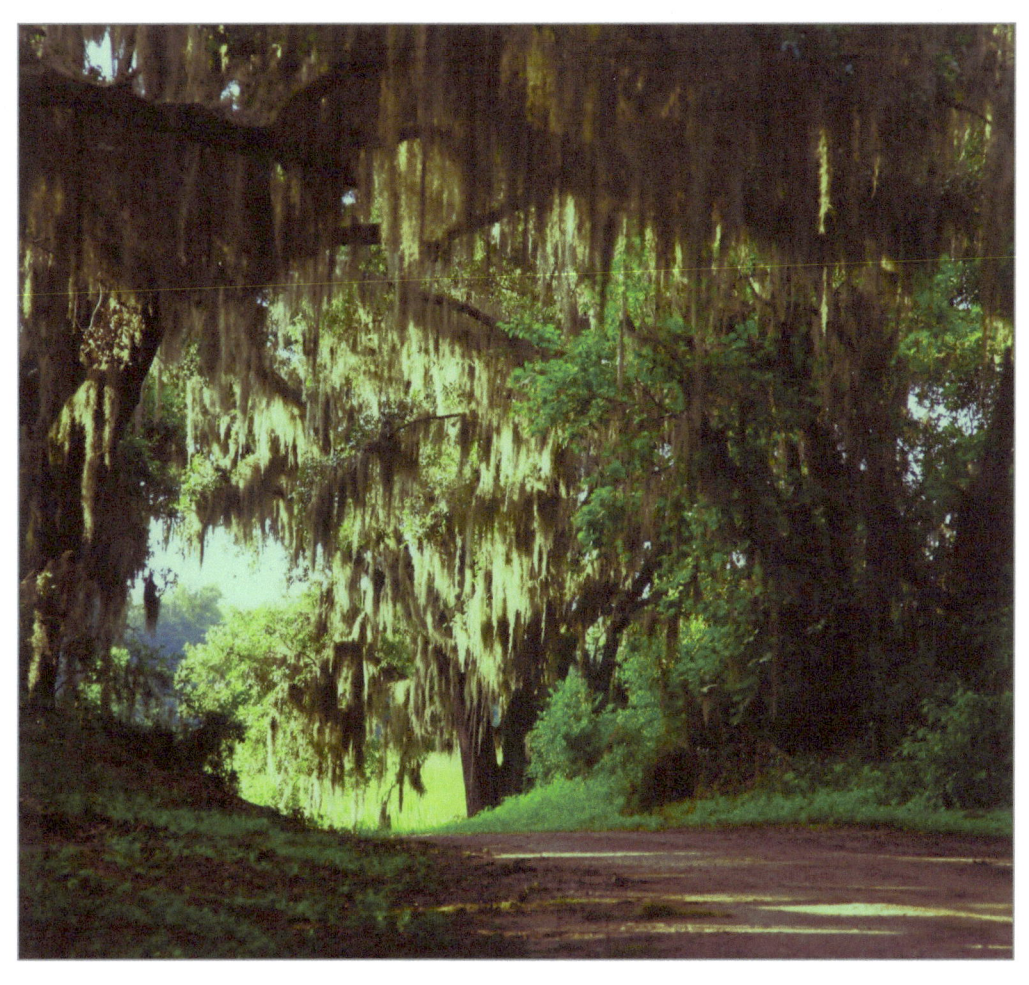

To be sure, I have no idea of the length, duration or destination of my journey with cancer. For many years I worked with children and teenagers who adopted an, "I Dunno" approach to the important questions of life. Today, I can sympathize with them as "I Dunno" where my trek is taking me or how it will end. But I am learning to be less afraid.

The thought occurs to me that this crisis in my life may be God's way of retooling me for a different purpose or direction. I think about automobile plants that periodically shut down for next year's model. I recall being retooled several times in my life. At one point, I loved working with the severely mentally ill. I preferred working with adults. But much of my career has centered on children and their families. I have training and experience working with prison inmates but found much of my work in this area focused on pre-delinquent teenagers. Each retooling has been fulfilling and beneficial.

Recently, I revisited the feeling of my lost identity due to my cancer. I am learning that my personal and professional identities are not the same. At this time in my life, my professional identity is blurred. But my personal identity is coming into focus. I continue working to maintain the validity of my "I love me" wall. Some might think this is an attempt at ego repair and maybe they are not altogether wrong. But I have learned how we label ourselves is very important to our quality of life. Am I now a "disabled person" or am I the "same person" fighting a serious life threatening disease? How we label ourselves shapes our lifestyles. I have learned we can choose our own labels.

Life has been good to me. I love life and frankly don't want to give it up. I am in no hurry to see my wife, mother, father, Aunt Tillly and Uncle Toad. Such a reunion may be wonderful but it is okay with me to put it off a while. I believe my loved ones will understand my reluctance. I consider life a gift of God's grace (unmerited favor). So no matter how my journey with cancer ends, perhaps I can learn to accept loss of life in the same spirit it was given.

David Schell © 2011

Clinically and statistically, I may not have long to live. But who knows the mind and will of God. Could it be the journey is as important as the destination? Should He retool me for a career change, I win. Should He restore my health and allow me to return to my practice, I win. Should He call me home, I win.

Time to Clean up: The Rotten Rat Syndrome

September, 2010

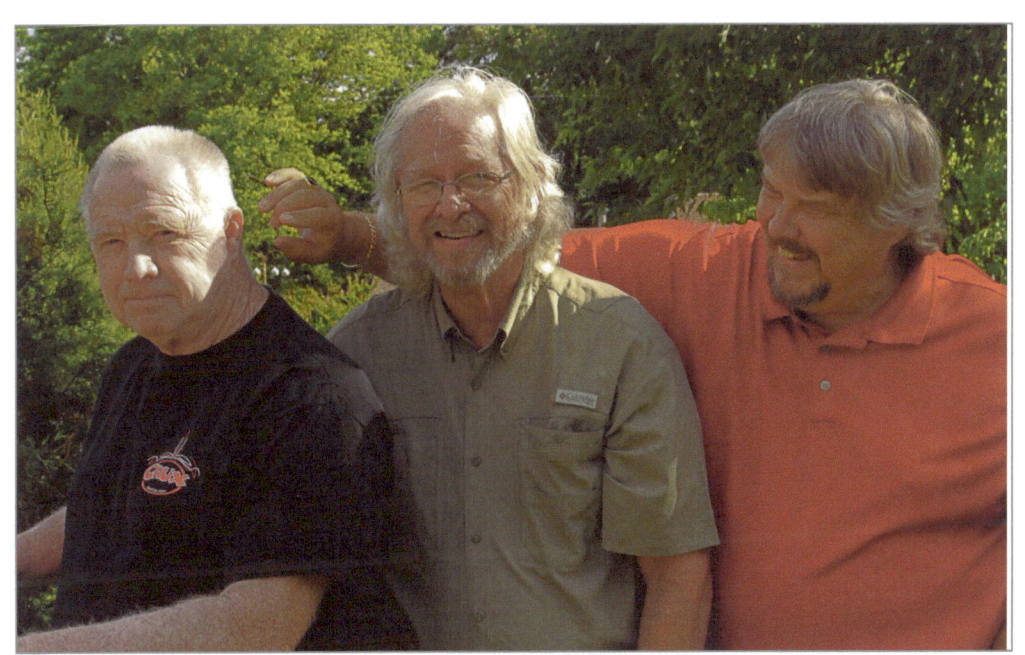

David Schell © 2011

Socrates taught that a life unexamined is not worth living. Certainly a round with cancer provides ample opportunity for self-examination. If we don't examine ourselves, we will certainly be examined and judged by others who may be less sympathetic.

I grew up in a home with two brothers and no sisters. We three brothers were pretty rough and tumble. Our mother was a very refined lady and experienced regular apoplexy over the behavior of her three crude little pigs. Like a lot of boys, we liked to play with rats and mice. Dead or alive, we could always use them to chase girls. During a large family Christmas celebration, one of my brothers came into the house reeking with a terribly foul odor. My mother was thoroughly embarrassed and quickly rushed him outside where she found several dead and decomposing rats in his jacket pocket. "Yup", it was time to clean up.

For over ten years I provided Mental Health Classroom Evaluations for Head Start classes which taught children ages 3-5. Of course during their activities, the children scattered toys and equipment all over the room. This was normal; creativity was encouraged. However, at the end of each module, the room had to be put back in order. The children were taught to chant, "Clean Up, Clean Up" as everything was put back into place in preparation for the next activity.

"Cancer" (Sometimes referred to as the Big C which sounds better than the real word) can serve as a clarion call to clean up our lives, situations, and circumstances. The very word "Cancer", much less a personal diagnosis, forces us to think about life and death issues. Of course, we are all destined to leave this world, so why not take a little time and put our best foot forward. This reminds me of ladies fixing their hair and putting on lipstick to go to Walmart. Sure can't hurt anything.

Internal bitterness, disbelief, feeling overwhelmed, anger, resentment and fear are common reactions to being told we have cancer. These feelings are normal but not comfortable or healthy and therefore need attention. Such feelings can soon turn into a pocket full of rotten rats.

My oncologist works hard adjusting my medications and dosages to assure I have the best quality of life possible and still maintain effective treatment against my cancer. This is a delicate balance that requires great skill. He reminds me many patients quit rather than endure ongoing treatment. I summon my courage and chose to continue.

In tandem with chemotherapy, it is my responsibility to achieve an inner quality of life. My oncologist and I talk freely about such a partnership. Spiritual, mental and emotional domains are generally my responsibilities. I have found cleansing myself of anger, hostility, resentment and malice, enhances the inner qualities of my life.

Emotionally and spiritually my saga with cancer has made me a better person. Even small vestures toward ridding myself of toxic thoughts, emotions and behaviors pay handsome dividends. I am not progressing toward sainthood or anything of that magnitude but am learning to experience a sense of inner peace in spite of the cancer. I feel a little more prepared for my journey home. Could it be that "Letting Go" is not so hard after all?

Even if our lives are extended into old age, an occasional personal assessment seems reasonable. On the other hand, should my cancer prove terminal, maybe I won't have to carry so much baggage.

I recall those painful days soon after surgery. My abdomen was bandaged with what seemed to be a very sticky tape. On one occasion that tape was quickly ripped off. I thought I had died and cried out, "I believe I am dead and things are not looking good on this side!" For a few minutes, I thought I had a near death experience. To use an old Southern expression, "That scared my mule".

Of course, one does not have to believe in an afterlife or adhere to any specific dogma to live with honor and dignity. Regardless of our beliefs and physical health, we can always be more loving, compassionate, caring and forgiving. We may never experience our "Fifteen Minutes in the Sun", but we can always create a meaningful legacy.

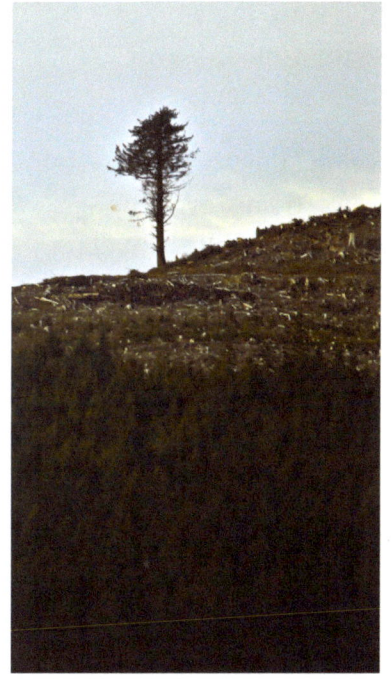

Earlier in my career a forty-year-old man with terminal cancer was referred to me along with his family. His doctors advised him he had less than a year to live. To be honest, I did not want the case. After all, he was terminal—not much chance of a success story here. (We therapists are not exempt from the tyranny of our own egos.) I soon found accepting this case would change my life more than his. I quickly came to admire and respect his inner strength and courage. Instead of being consumed by anger, he began preparing himself and his family. This family would never regret failing to express their love for one another.

Yet, tragedy continued to haunt this man. During the year he had left, his wife suddenly died. A few weeks later his son was killed in an accident. Nevertheless, the last few months of his life were a monument to the human spirit of love and courage. He inspired all who had the privilege of knowing him. In spite of my credentials posted on my "I Love Me Wall", he was the therapist, I was the client. Did he get his fifteen minutes in the sun? Not really, but he changed my life and attitude regarding the remaining years of my practice.

My saga with cancer and pursuit of personal adjustment has been something like a merry-go-round. Merry-go-rounds are designed for fun, but everyone has to pay to ride. Unfortunately, merry-go-rounds can also create motion sickness. Some rides are stationary and stable while others go up and down and can make us aware of the hot dogs and cotton candy we ate before climbing aboard. Of course there is always hope of the elusive brass ring.

David Schell © 2011

No matter how rough our journey with cancer becomes, we can always be better people.

Not long ago I read Mother Theresa had confessed she spent many years feeling lonely, dry and tortured in spite of her beautiful and loving accomplishments. I wondered if she had not carried a rotten rat a little too long. But who am I to judge? Her life's journey was far more complicated than mine. Maybe like Mother Theresa, in spite of obstacles, we can keep on keeping on.

For starters, we can learn to clean our closets by forgiving others and ourselves. We can learn to accept, appreciate and love ourselves for "trying" even though reaching perfection is not a reasonable goal. Forgiveness turns lose a lot of rotten rats.

The world loved Mother Theresa for the quality of her trying, not for attaining perfection. With that in mind I strongly suspect there is hope for the rest of us. Maybe within the scope of our personal cancer journeys, we can someday say, "Been there, done that, and got the Tee-shirt".

Several years ago, I had a fifteen-year-old young lady as a client who suffered a rare and painful terminal disease. Repeated surgeries extended her life but only for short periods of time. During one of her stays at a university hospital, a doctor attempted to explain to her what "terminal" meant. (I have been in similar situations and profoundly appreciate the difficulty of his task.) He began by asking my young client if she knew the meaning of "terminal". With determination she rose to the occasion and exclaimed, "Of course I know what it means to be terminal! We are ALL terminal!" I was honored to share that incident at her funeral.

At some point, all of us, cancer or not, are going to "kick the bucket" or "push up daisies" or in more refined terms, "God will call us home". These are some of the many euphemisms for death. We can dance around reality, but reality is always there. I learned from my young client I could choose to live with my cancer or spend the rest of my life dying from it. We are all terminal.

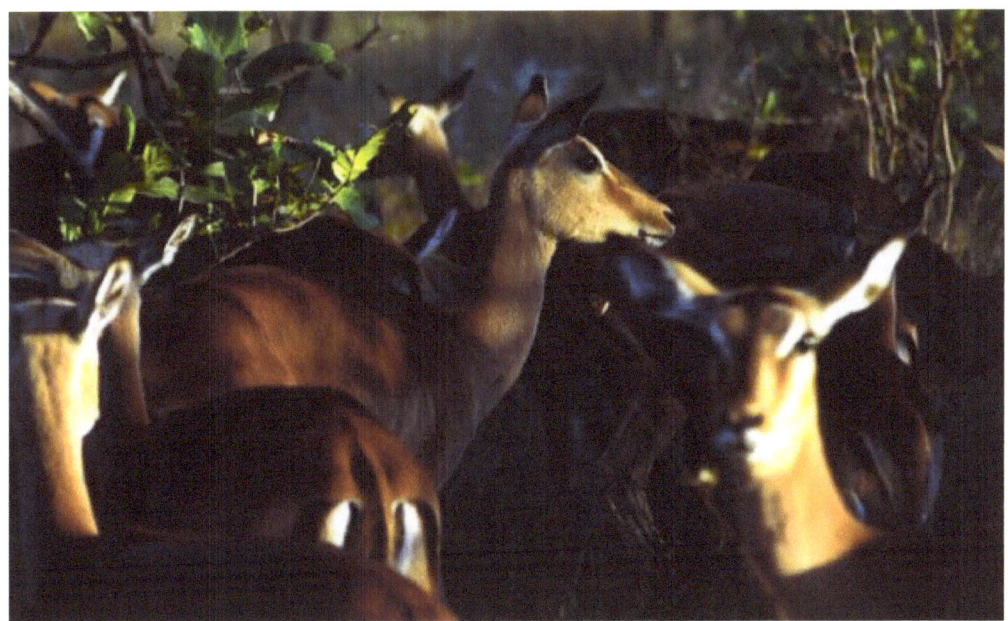

Most cultures and religions teach judgment follows death. For instance, the ancient Egyptians developed a very systematic concept of judgment. Now we are getting into scary stuff. For some of us, it is scarier than for others. I recall the story of two little boys whose grandmother stopped baking cookies and started reading her Bible for hours every day. Their mother sensed their concern and confided, "Don't worry; Grandma is just catching up on her homework".

Since no one can clinically "prove" the existence of God, much less His methods of judgment let me share some thoughts that have been helpful to me. Not everyone believes in the existence of God which does not mean they don't have inner spiritual resources. On the other hand, most Americans believe in God though their beliefs are varied. The basic conundrum is that God exists or He does not exist. Either way can be ominous. If there is no God, the world seems to be running amok and no one is in control. If there is a God, we may be answerable to Him.

I suspect God judges us on the basis of our trying and efforts to show love to our fellowman rather than our failures. Human law judges primarily on actual behaviors with the possible exception of conspiracies which also have their behavioral components. God's judgment may focus on intentions of the heart rather than the outcome of our failures. For instance, a couple of years ago, I failed to yield the right of way to a car I did not see. I did not mean to cause an accident. Putting others and myself in danger was not my intention. My intention was to turn safely into traffic. Yet, due to my behavior I caused and was charged with the accident. I would like to have been judged by my intentions. The legal system rarely looks on the heart. Though I can't speak for God, I think He ALWAYS looks on the heart.

Certainly, much of our aberrant behavior is related to personal choices. Several years ago, I wrote a book titled: Getting Bitter or Getting Better: Choosing Forgiveness for Your Own Good. I stressed choice implies control and leaves a lot of room for individual growth and development. After the book was published, my father read it. Closing the book, he succinctly summarized, "Life is what you make it". My father was a very wise man. By the way, forgiveness may also lead to compassion for others who are also subject to human failures. Mother Theresa's life was an example of such compassion.

Ever think of shopping for a religion that does not believe in judgment? Can't say it hasn't crossed my mind.

LETTING GO AND REACHING OUT

OCTOBER, 2010

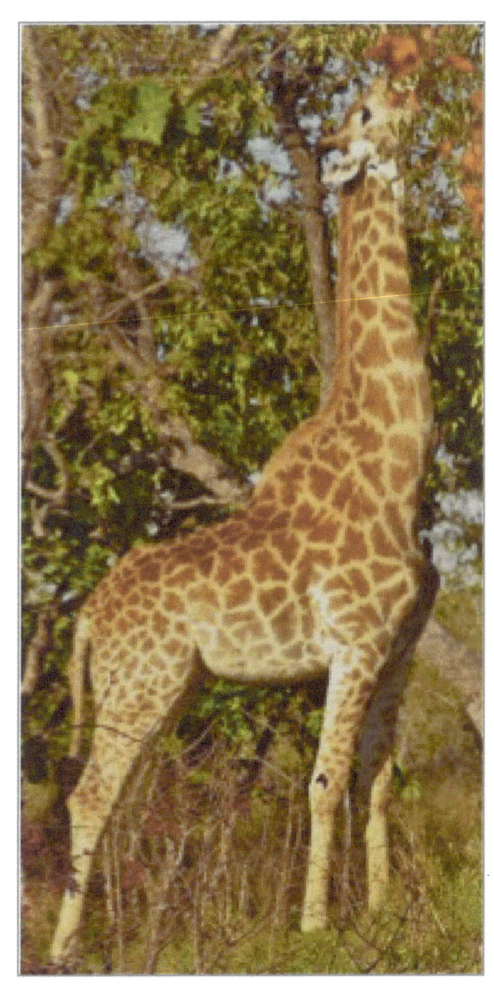

I am one who needs a lot of prayer. I am often reminded of a preacher friend of mine who quipped, "David, pray for me. I need the prayer; you need the practice". No debate there. In truth, I am one who needs both prayer and practice. Of course not everyone falls into my category. I know many wonderful people for whom a simple, "Now I lay me down to sleep" is perfectly sufficient.

For me, prayer is expressing my hopes and concerns to God. I don't worry about His hearing my prayers. I leave that up to Him. I don't worry about His answering my prayers. Again, I leave that up to Him. I think that constitutes at least a modicum of faith.

I view myself as a person with at least a thread of faith. I see others who seem to have fully woven tapestries. Sometimes it is hard for me to hold onto my thread. To paraphrase Socrates, an unexamined faith is not worth living. A questioned faith can be a tempered faith.

Certainly a journey through the perils of cancer can either dash our hopes or strengthen our faith. That part is left up to us. The question comes to me, "When is it time to let go and reach out?" Cancer is a major crisis in my life. It is potentially lethal. I can't throw it off casually. My inquisitive mind wrestles with further questions: Letting go of what? Reaching out for what? Does letting go diminish my autonomy? Does letting go create an unnecessary dependence? To be sure, resources surround me. These resources include: the medical community, family, friends, prayer groups, and ultimately, in my view, our Creator. But the question remains, "When is it time to let go and reach out?"

Three year old children are often heard to say, "I can do it by myself". They are learning independence and autonomy. In many ways I find myself fixated at this stage of development. Fearing the loss of independence and autonomy, many of us have a hard time reaching out. We may feel it as a loss of our personal integrity. Sometimes my little three-year-old inner child can be such a tyrant.

Having experienced times of total helplessness, I have finally concluded it is appropriate to reach out when problems and circumstances are BIGGER than we are. Stage 4 cancer is bigger than I am. I need help. Reaching out at such times does not diminish us as autonomous human beings, rather it affirms our humanity. I have also discovered reaching out can also strengthen our friends who long to help us.

Reaching out can be a slippery slope. What if I fall into the abyss of dependency? Dependency can become a lifestyle. Dependency can be used to manipulate others to do our bidding. This type of dependency frequently deteriorates relationships and risks creating resentment among caregivers. Disabled people can become tyrants. Will reaching out provide the safety net I need? Will my reluctance to reach out cast me into a prison of loneliness? How will my decisions affect my voyage with cancer? These are all important questions, but the bottom line is I need help when I need help.

Professionals in my field often make the distinction between "enabling" and "empowerment". Enabling clients by doing "for" them is much different than empowering them by doing "with" them. Empowerment is designed to maximize one's own inner resources and learn to function effectively beyond the therapist's office. Enabling clients only fosters dependence; empowerment provides needed strength. For years the major goal for most of my clients was to put myself out of business with them. I worked hard to avoid crippling them with dependence. Yet, some clients struggle with problems of such magnitude, they must learn to reach out when necessary. I call to mind children and adults who are severely mentally impaired. Cancer can and does impair some individuals to the extent they cannot function. Sometimes, dependency cannot be avoided.

Yes, there are times when I must let go of my pride and reach out to those who love me or have the skills to prolong or enhance the quality of my life. To be sure cancer remains bigger than I am and could bring about my demise. I cannot rationally avoid reaching out. Yet, God seems to give me strength to do many things for myself.

Though I am not in active practice at this time, people often come to me with concerns for their families or children. Recently, while attached to an infusion tube in the clinic, I held three informal unplanned sessions with individuals who reported being significantly helped. In truth, I was helped most of all. He restoreth my dignity.

Good News;
Bad News
And a Whole Lot
in Between

January, 2011

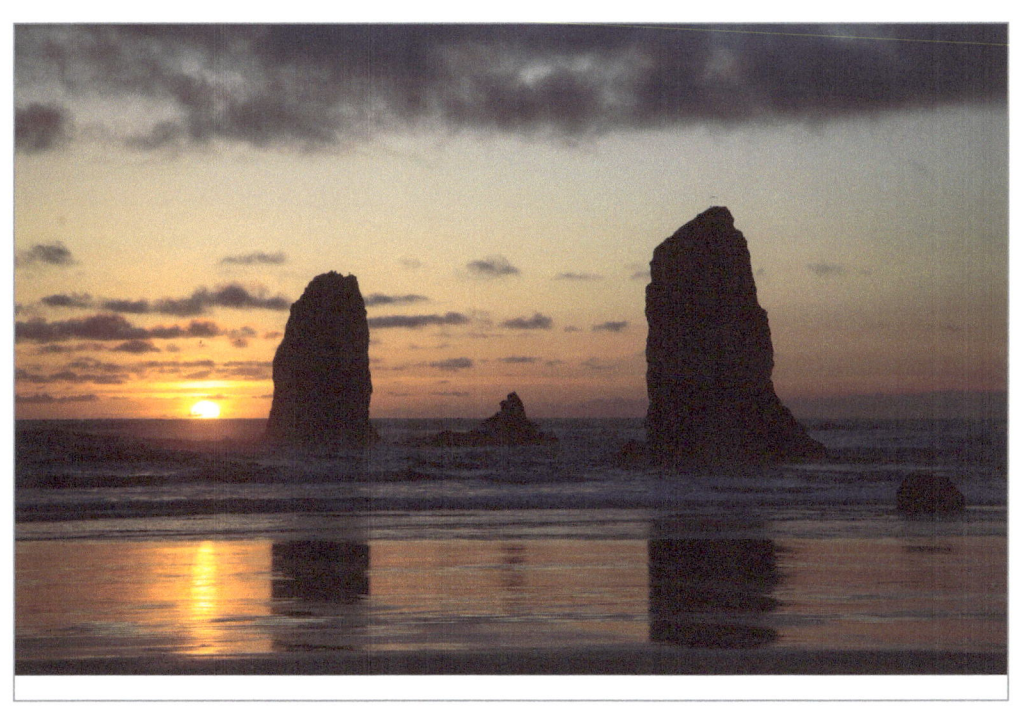

Good News: I am still here.

Bad News: The ultimate destiny of my cancer journey is still vague. Sometimes, I feel like an abandoned pirate ship floating aimlessly on the high seas. Nevertheless, reviewing cancer related events and feelings over the past year has helped me take a more objective and realistic assessment of my life and circumstances. For instance, I have experienced some major accomplishments in my own spiritual and emotional journey. I have also been able to help others who are struggling with difficult life circumstances. However, I am still unable to resume my professional practice.

In my quest to make sense of my journey, I found it helpful to list some Good News/Bad News situations that have occurred over the past year. Good News: I have given a few talks on coping with cancer and have a professional presentation on the subject scheduled in the near future. Bad News: I am weakened and must lecture while seated in a chair. Good News: I feel good most days. Bad News: Some days I feel like absolute crap. Good News: I have met many wonderful cancer victims and helping professionals. Bad News: I have to go to the cancer clinic to see most of them. Good News: I have seen others cured of cancer. Bad News: I still have mine.

I recall, when my cancer and lymphoma were first diagnosed, I was told without treatment I might have about six more months to live. A year later, I am alive and having a lot of good days. A cure does not seem to be on the horizon, but who knows the mind of God. At my age, I don't expect a major "cure-all" in my lifetime. In the meantime, I continue receiving the best care available. Some days the chemotherapy makes me sick. On those bad days I have learned to thank God, as feeling bad is also a signal the medication is eating away at my cancer.

Early in my journey, someone suggested the Lord has prepared a mansion for me somewhere in the great beyond. I recalled the primary rule in real estate is location, location, location. A year has passed and apparently my loan has not yet been approved.

I am not sure when my cancer began. It was advanced by the time it was discovered. I was diagnosed in January 2010. So I have chosen that date as my mark in time. This gives me extra reasons to celebrate Christmas and New Year's.

Just before Christmas my urine began showing proteins that should not be there and which threatened permanent damage to my kidneys. I was given a big red half-gallon jug and ordered to collect urine for the next twenty-four hours and bring it to the laboratory the next day. I dutifully peed in the jug as instructed. The next day I attached a large Christmas bow to the jug and took it back to the clinic and laboratory. All professionalism fell apart. I have come to love those people and feel pretty sure they love me too. I have found such love is emotionally and spiritually healing. Good News: I am surrounded by love. Bad News: I need to be more loving.

People like William James, Norman Vincent Peale, and Albert Ellis, each very different than the others have taught us our thinking, feeling and behavior are interconnected and can be controlled by the individual. I used to direct an alcohol and drug detoxification ward where we often said, "It is the stinkin' thinkin' that causes the drinkin'". Of course, bad thinking can cause more than drinking. The good news is that we can change our thinking and it will change our feelings and behavior. We can change anyone of the three and with a little effort the other two will also change. James indicated this was one of the major discoveries in his century.

These men challenge us to take control of our thinking, feeling, and behavior. I associate these changes with attitude. Good News: I can control my attitude regarding my journey with cancer. Bad News: Sometimes I don't.

Feelings of desolation and discouragement are normal but not comfortable. Good News: I have learned negative feelings can be controlled. Controlling my feelings is not necessarily easy but the choice is largely up to me. Bad News: Sometimes I forget I can control my thinking, feelings and behavior.

I think back over the past year and recall my initial reaction, "Holy cow, I have cancer! Now what?" Today, I still have cancer, but I am learning to let go and come to peace with it. Not all my, "Now what?" questions are answered but I have come to believe while we are on earth, the journey is more important than the destination. Cancer can serve to slow us down so we can enjoy the beauty and rich qualities of life all around us. The love and support of family and friends are treasures beyond measure. One can learn to savor each moment and decide what is really important in life.

I ponder, is this idea of "Letting Go and Letting God…" a perfect answer? No. No more than I am a perfect human being. I am not exempt from frustration and desolation. However, practicing this concept has proven to be marvelous therapy for me. Yes, some days I feel frustration and desolation al a mode. But most days, I just enjoy the ice cream.

> *- David W. Schell, Ed.D.*
> *April, 2011*

"Should God be willin' and the crick don't rise," to be continued. . .

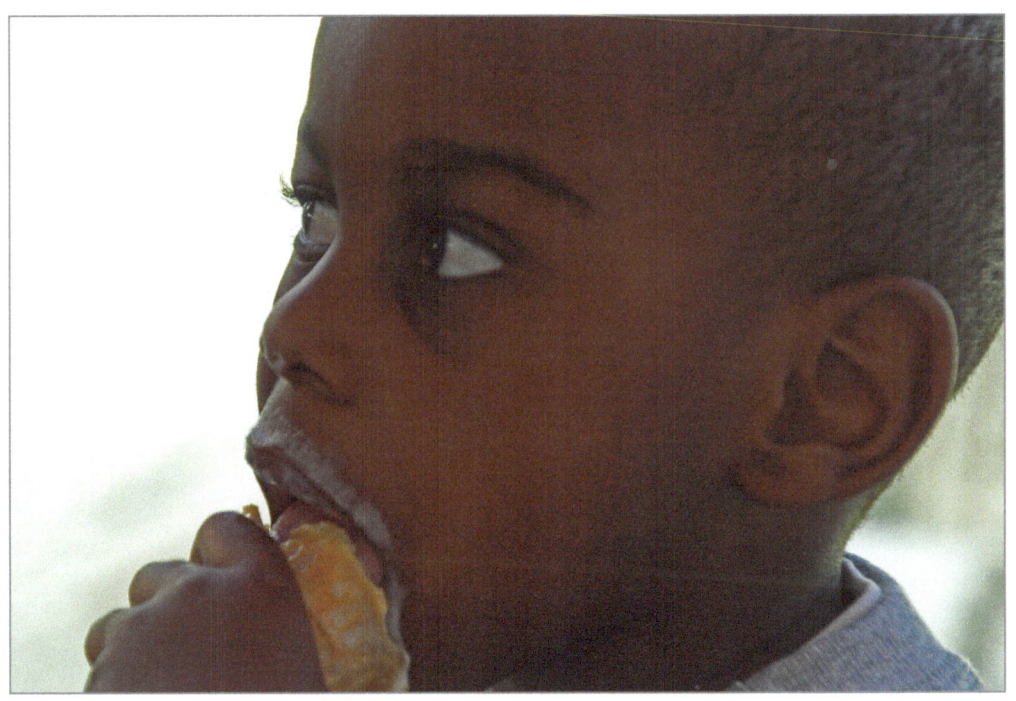

POSTSCRIPT

I don't suppose many books have gone to press without the author wishing certain passages had been included. I am sure that will be the case with this book as well. However, I cannot close this book without mentioning that we three rough and tumble Schell Boys have each been stricken with widely diverse types of Cancer. My brother, Daniel, expresses our concerns so well, before closing this book; I must share his reflections with you:

"I was asked by my brother, David, if I would contribute to his manuscript on cancer and his journey with this disease. Of course, I was more than happy to do so."I too, have heard my doctor use the dreaded C word. I remember when we were boys our parents warned us not to use certain the four letter words. Today I think the four letter words have been replaced by a six letter word, CANCER.

Although my cancer was diagnosed as skin cancer it is something nobody wants to hear. Fortunately mine was Basil Cell Carcinoma, not Melanoma. Thank God! I watched my father-in-law die from cancer. He fought it for over seven years. His too started with skin cancer.

Mine started as a small lesion on my right arm just above the wrist that wouldn't heal. I went to my regular medical doctor and was told not to worry about it and was given an ointment. Three months later I went back to the same doctor. At that time, I was told that the place was not healing because of my diabetes and was put on an antibiotic. However, the lesion did not change. Four months later I went to a dermatologist and was told that my hands and arms were the worst ones she had ever seen. She immediately froze over thirty spots, biopsied four places including the lesion and made an appointment have the large one removed.

By the time it was removed it was approximately the size of the bottom of a Styrofoam coffee cup. Within a month I had four cancers removed from my right arm. I have just completed four PDF light treatments on both arms.

I can't emphasize enough the importance of early detection by an oncologist or a dermatologist. I hope that by reading this book and sharing our experiences, a life may be saved or someone can be cured by early detection and treatment. I believe that the right care and the power of prayer have helped me. I pray every day for my brothers, David and John.

I sincerely hope that this will reach and help someone. Cancer not only affects the person who has it but also affects all who love and care about them."

- D.R. Schell

Further along we'll know all about it ...

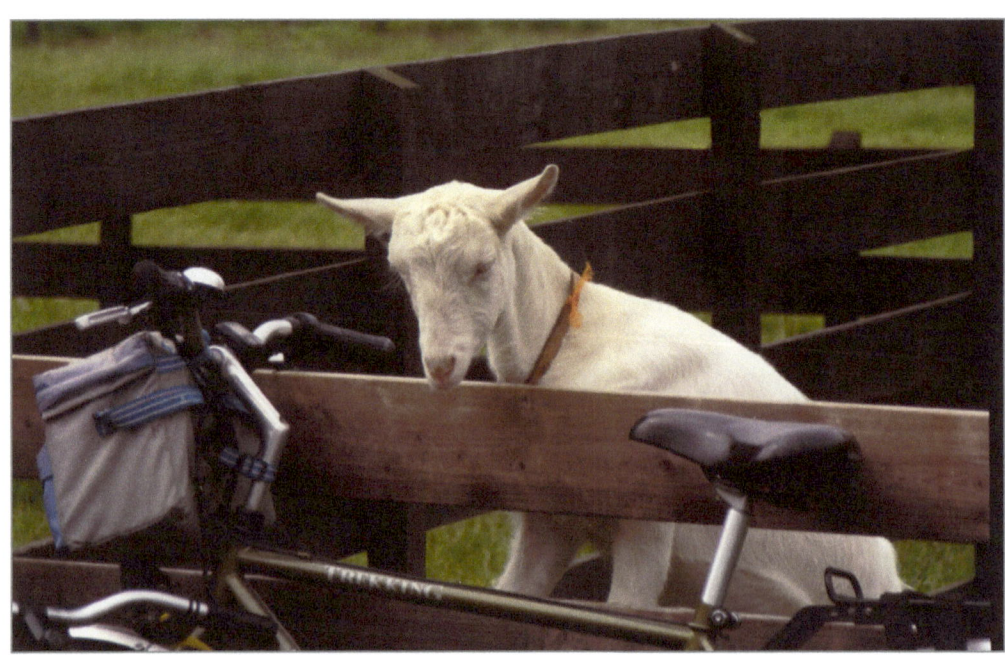

Holy Cow! I Have CANCER! Now What?